How To Relieve Neck Pain And Avoid Neck Surgery

A Step-By-Step Guide Put Together by the Clinic Director of the Back Pain And Sciatica Clinic in Soquel, CA

DR. JOHN FALKENROTH, D.C.

DEDICATION

This is dedicated to the countless number of people in this world who suffer from neck pain. I hope that this material that I put together will help neck pain sufferers get neck pain relief.

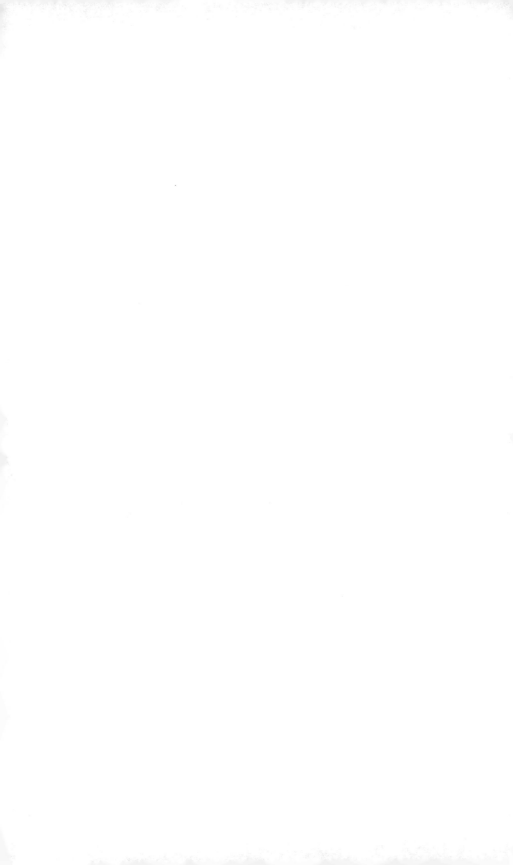

CONTENTS

	Acknowledgments	i
	Special Note	ii
1	The 6 Common Causes Of Neck Pain	1 - 5
2	Can Your Neck Pain Come From Other Places Besides Your Neck And Head?	6 - 7
3	How To Sleep When Your Neck Hurts	8 - 10
4	How To Determine If Your Headache Is Coming From A Problem In Your Neck	11 - 12
5	What Is A "Slipped Disc" Or A Herniated Disc In The Neck?	13 - 15
6	How Neck Pain Usually Starts And How It Gets Worse	16 - 20
7	What You Should Avoid When Your Neck Hurts	21 - 25
8	The Proper Standing And Sitting Posture For Neck Pain Relief	26 - 30
9	Walk … Walk… Walk…	31 - 33
10	How Much Water You Should Drink For Your Condition	34 - 35
11	Should You Use Ice Or Heat For Your Neck Pain?	36 - 37
12	Neck Pain Exercises That You Should Consider Doing	38 - 45
13	How To Keep Your Spine Aligned And Moving Properly	46 - 49
14	Neck Pain Treatment Options	50 - 56

ACKNOWLEDGMENTS

Thank you to all of my patients who have given me the privilege of trusting me with their health.

Thank you also to the thousands of patients who listened to my guidance. They have helped me gain the knowledge and the experience to further help others who suffer from back pain, neck pain and sciatica.

Thank you to all of the wonderful teachers throughout my life who gave me a solid educational foundation and instilled in me the love of learning.

Finally, I'd like to thank my family – my wife Estrella and my children James, Kevin and Starlyn – for their love and support.

SPECIAL NOTE

The information contained in this guide is solely advisory, and should not be substituted for medical advice. Any and all health care concerns, decisions, and actions must be done through the advice and counsel of a healthcare professional who is familiar with your updated medical history. We cannot be held responsible for actions you may take without a thorough exam or appropriate referral. If your condition is so severe that you have symptoms that prompt immediate surgical consideration such as loss of bladder and/or bowel control, etc., please get immediate medical care for your condition. Also understand that your results will vary. By following the information contained in this guide, you realize that you are doing so at your own risk and knowingly waive all rights to make any legal claims against Dr. John Falkenroth, D.C. or Back Pain & Sciatica Clinic or any site and/or site affiliates that this information may appear on.

1 THE 6 COMMON CAUSES OF NECK PAIN

Up to 70% of the general population will have neck pain at some point in their life. Recovery within the year from neck pain ranges between 33% and 65%... AND relapses are common throughout the lifetime of the neck pain patient.

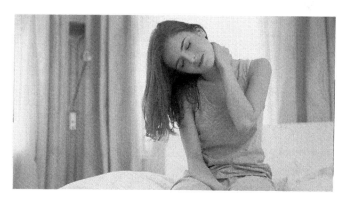

In general, neck pain is more common in women,
higher in high-income countries, and higher in urban regions.
The greatest risk for neck pain occurs between 35 - 49 years of age.

Neck pain is a very common problem that can come from a lot of places. It can come from laying crooked while watching TV, it can come from sleeping the wrong way, it can arise from an injury like car accidents, it can come from overlifting or carrying and it can come from pinching the phone between your ear and shoulder.

1

You may also experience neck pain as a response to a cold or a flu... also your neck can hurt because of a referred pain from a sinus infection.

Neck pain can even come from "stress." Rare but dangerous causes of neck pain include bleeding inside the head during a stroke… or neck pain due to a heart attack. For these two rare causes of neck pain, you must get emergency care right away.

There is even a category of causation called "insidious" or "idiopathic" which means we DON'T KNOW where the neck pain is coming from.

It's important to understand that neck pain is a symptom… not a disease… which means we have to identify the cause...if we can. This is why a detailed evaluation is required.

Below are 6 common causes of neck pain:

1.) MUSCLES: There are MANY layers of muscles in the neck. There are very small, deep muscles that are important for stability of the spine. There are larger outside muscles that are long and strong, allowing us to sustain stresses like playing football, rugby, hockey, or falling on the ice.

Bad posture, long car drives/rides, computer work, studying/reading, or having a conversation with someone not sitting directly in front of you are just a few examples of how these muscles can experience overuse that can generate neck pain.

2.) LIGAMENTS: These are tough, non-stretching tissues that hold bone to bone and can tear in trauma like car accident or whiplash, while playing sports, or in a fall.

Because ligaments are important in keeping our joints stable, disrupted ligaments can lead to excessive sliding back and forth of our neck bones when we move our neck.

This can wear down the cartilage or the smooth, silky covering at the ends of bones. This can lead to premature arthritis called osteoarthritis.

3) WORN JOINTS: As we age, our joints will degenerate. In the neck, there are two sets of small joints between six of the seven vertebrae called facet joints and uncinate processes that are vulnerable to osteoarthritis. Arthritis in your neck can create bone spurs than can pinch your nerve. (see

2

#5 below). Because of this, arthritic joints are frequent neck pain generators. If you hear noise in your neck when you move it, your neck joints might be starting to wear down and get arthritic.

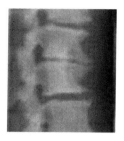

**Here's an example of what worn arthritic joints
with bone spurs look like in the spine.**

The most common cause of arthritic spinal joints is repetitive microinjuries to your spine... such as sitting for a long time, improper posture, incorrect spinal biomechanics when lifting, improper spinal motion... and uncorrected spinal misalignments.

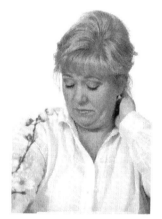

**Sitting at a desk for a long time
without taking frequent breaks
can result in degeneration of your neck joints.**

4) DISC INJURY: Over time (years), repeated injuries to the neck can result in Degenerative Disc Disease. These small discs lose their water retaining capabilities... and become narrow and less flexible... which is a common source of neck pain and stiffness.

3

The discs rest between the big vertebral bodies and act as shock absorbers. They are like jelly donuts, and when the disc's tough outer layers tear, the jelly can leak out and this may or may not hurt, depending on the direction, the amount of the leaked out "jelly," and if the "jelly" pinches pain-sensitive tissues. A "herniated disc" is the most common cause of a pinched nerve (see #5 below). A herniated disc in your neck can also cause "referred pain" in your shoulder blade.

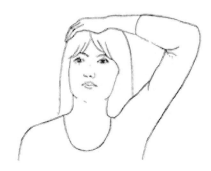

**This position can help you determine
if you have a herniated disc in your neck.**

If you have the <u>CLASSIC</u> presentation of a patient with a herniated disc in the neck, here's what you'll experience:

When you hold your arm over your head, you'll find relief. This is because this position puts slack in your nerve and it hurts less in this position. Also, you'll notice that looking up usually hurts more... and can increase your arm or hand pain/numbness... while looking down reduces your symptoms.

5) <u>NERVE COMPRESSION:</u> The nerves in your neck travel to your arms. Your nerve can be compressed or pinched by a bulged disc, herniated disc, bone spur, excessive ligament thickness, tumor or cyst. Any of these can lead to narrowing of the hole where the pinched nerve exits... a condition known as spinal stenosis.

Nerve compression or pinching of a nerve can result in numbness or tingling or burning pain in your arm and/or hand and/or shoulder. Your symptoms may affect one or both sides. Your arms and hands may also feel weaker. In the early stages, this shows up as clumsiness or dropping things from your hand.

Each nerve has a different role. Mapping the numbness area and testing your reflexes and muscle strength... can help us identify your specific nerve that is injured.

6)   DISEASES: Though less common, neck pain can be caused by certain diseases such as rheumatoid arthritis, meningitis and/or cancer. When these are suspect, blood tests and special tests such as bone scan, CT/MRI, and/or biopsy can help to specifically identify your condition. Also, as mentioned earlier, neck pain can also be caused by stroke or heart attack.

2 CAN YOUR NECK PAIN COME FROM OTHER PLACES BESIDES YOUR NECK AND HEAD?

Neck pain and stiffness are very common complaints, and these problems can come and go chronically for years, even decades. Focusing ONLY on the neck may NOT be the best approach. Here's why...

A group of physical therapists in Brazil and Australia performed a systematic literature review of the benefits of specific stabilization exercises for spinal and pelvic pain and looked at disability, return to work, number of episodes, global perceived benefit, and quality of life factors.

They not only searched for the beneficial effects for low back and pelvic pain and dysfunction... but also the benefits for headache with or without neck pain and any related disability.

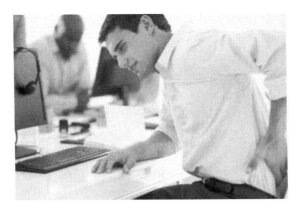

Can your neck pain be coming from your low back?

Their study found significant research support for improving pelvic pain and for preventing recurrence after an acute episode of low back pain. But, they also found that cervicogenic headache and neck pain improved from the use of low back/pelvic stabilization exercises. Cervicogenic headache is headache caused by problems in the neck.

These findings suggest that stabilizing your low back and pelvis may help relieve your neck pain. How? A stable low back and pelvis offers the neck and head a better foundation on which to rest. An analogy would be a house with a weak foundation resulting in the whole house being unstable, especially the attic or the area farthest away from the ground.

Since improving the stability of the low back and pelvis helped relieve neck pain, maybe some neck pain may be caused by problems in the low back and/or pelvis.

3 HOW TO SLEEP WHEN YOUR NECK HURTS

If you've ever had neck pain, then you already know how challenging it is to find a comfortable position in bed and how difficult it can be to fall asleep and stay asleep. In fact, sometimes neck pain can get so bad, that lying down is not even an option.

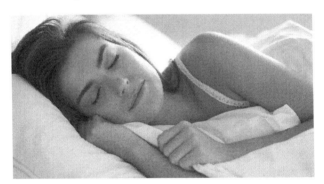

**Sleep… especially deep sleep…
is a VERY important part of healing your neck pain.**

A Harvard based report states that 75% of us get less than 6 hours of sleep at least a few nights per week. Over the short haul, this is not a problem. But, in the long haul, this is a BIG PROBLEM.

The report lists "Six reasons not to skimp on sleep:"

1. Learning and memory – "memory consolidation" occurs better after we sleep when learning new tasks and test scores reflect the difference

2. Weight and metabolism – chronic sleep problems can cause weight gain by altering the way our body processes and stores carbohydrates and by altering the hormones that affect appetite

3. Safety – lack of sleep results in increased fatigue, which in turn results in a greater tendency to fall asleep during the day. This can be catastrophic such as in car accidents, industrial accidents, etc.

4. Mood – the lack of sleep can increase irritability, impatience, concentration loss and moodiness

5. Heart health – serious sleep loss has been linked to hypertension, increased stress hormone levels, and irregular heartbeat

6. Disease – sleep problem alters immune function and sleeping well may help fight cancer

So now that you know the benefits of good sleep, how can you sleep well when your neck hurts?

As a start, avoid caffeine at least 2-3 hours before bedtime. Also, for some, exercising too close to bedtime is not helpful.

Regarding neck posture while sleeping, the proper pillow is VERY IMPORTANT. Try lying on your back and both sides… but preferably not your stomach due to the need to rotate the neck when you lie on your stomach.

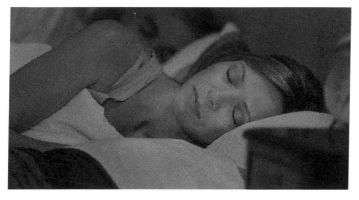

Use a pillow that's not too thick or too thin.

The "ideal pillow" is one that allows your neck to remain "neutral" or maintain its proper normal curve that is present when you're standing.

Since our neck is generally skinnier than our head, a "neck-friendly" pillow should be thicker on the edge... so that it fills in the space between the neck and the bed... and thinner under the head. This is true whether we lay on our sides or back, but the amount of space varies with age, gender, and phenotype – that is, thin, medium or heavy-set body types.

There are many contoured or "shaped" pillows available that are thicker on the outside edges and thinner in the middle. Some of these include foam pillows of different densities, air pillows, water pillows, memory foam pillows, feather pillows, and others.

Some companies make a pillow based on the measurement between the neck and the point of the shoulder. This allows the person to pick the pillow size best suited for their neck size. It's important to note that it can take about a week to get used to the "new shaped" pillow, so "BE PATIENT."

Since we spend 6-8 hours in bed sleeping... that's 25-30% of our life is spent sleeping... it's very important to sleep with your neck in good position. Also, keep in mind that it's easier to get used to a new pillow when you don't hurt, so may want to try a new pillow when your neck pain is not severe and you're feeling good.

4 HOW TO DETERMINE IF YOUR HEADACHE IS COMING FROM A PROBLEM IN YOUR NECK

Among the many types of headaches, one very common type is called the "cervicogenic headache."

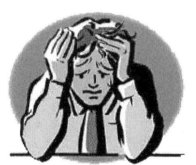

**A cervicogenic headache is
caused by a problem in your neck.**

There are 7 bones in your neck and 8 pairs of nerves that exit these bones and go to your head, neck, shoulders, arms, and fingers.

Think of your nerves as electric wires that stretch between a switch and a light bulb. The place where each nerve exits your neck bone is the switch and the target it travels to is the light bulb. If one were to stimulate each of the nerves as they exit the neck bones, we could "map" exactly where each nerve travels. This has been done.

11

When we look at the upper 3 sets of nerves that exit the neck, we see that as soon as they exit, right away they go up into the head (the scalp). Like any nerve, if enough pressure is applied to the nerve, the nerve gets damaged and you'll notice sensations like pain, tingling, numbness, burning or weakness.

If the pressure stays, these symptoms can last for a long time. So if you have a pinched nerve in your upper neck, you can get headaches.

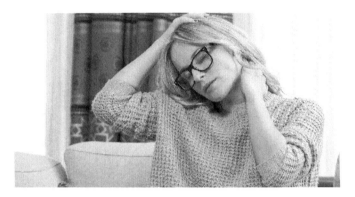

**One way to tell if your headache
is coming from your neck is to move your neck.**

If when you move your neck you start to get a headache… or if the headache you already have gets worse… then your headache is most likely coming from a problem in your neck.

Also, take a look in the mirror. Does your head tilt to one side? Does your head stick out in front of you instead of sitting back over your shoulders? These bad postures/positions can negatively affect your neck muscles and joints and cause headaches.

If your headache is coming from a problem in your neck, spinal treatments of the upper part of your neck can help relieve your headaches and your neck pain.

5 WHAT EXACTLY IS A "SLIPPED DISC" OR A HERNIATED DISC IN THE NECK?

When someone tells you that you have a cervical disc problem or a herniated disc, do you know what that means? The term "cervical" means neck. The term "disc" refers to the shock absorbing fibro-elastic cartilage that rests between each vertebra of the spine.

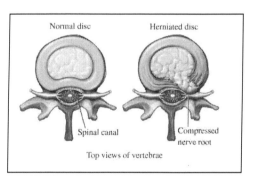

Think of the disc as being similar to a jelly donut.

The center of the disc is liquid-like - kind of like petroleum jelly. The outer part is tough and strong and circles the center like the rings of a freshly cut oak tree stump... its job is to hold the jelly-like part in the center of the disc.

What makes the outer layer so strong is the type of tissue it's made up of and, maybe most important, the opposing criss-cross pattern of each layer or ring of the annulus. Studies have shown that when the disc is pierced with a knife and then compressed, this criss-cross pattern of the annulus layers self-seals the cut, resulting in no leakage of the liquid center. You're probably wondering… how can a disc rupture, herniate or "slip" if it's so tough, strong, and self-sealing?

The answer: as the disc ages or when it's injured, tears or "fissures" in the disc fibers occur creating channels for the liquid part to work its way out towards the edge and eventually break through the outermost layer – hence, the term "herniated disc." It's similar to stepping on that jelly donut until the jelly leaks out to the point where you can see it.

Here's the strange part. Research tells us that about 50% of people have bulging discs (not quite herniated through) and 20% of us have herniated discs (that have popped through) but have NO PAIN AT ALL!

That makes it tough since an MRI or CT scan may show a herniated or bulging disc but how do we know that's the disc that's clinically important – the one that's creating the pain? That's why I treat patients and not their image (MRI, CT scan or x-ray).

Even though a disc may be bulging or herniated, I may not necessarily treat that particular disc if it's not expressing a problem clinically. A herniated disc in the neck creates a shooting pain down your arm and/or hands - usually below the elbow often into either the thumb or pinky side of the hand. You may have abnormal reflexes and abnormal sensation.

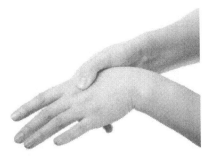

If you have a herniated disc in your neck,
your arms and hands may feel weaker.
In the early stages, this shows up as clumsiness –
for example, you may drop things from your hand.

Depending on which nerve(s) get irritated, problems can include

14

headaches, fainting, light-headedness, dizziness, shoulder blade pain, arm and/or hand pain, numbness and/or weakness.

You may also develop muscle spasms. This is due to a reflex reaction where the brain receives the pain signals from the neck and in response, sends signals back to the muscles to tighten in attempt to protect the problem.

This becomes a "vicious cycle" and may continue until the problematic joint is unlocked or released… or until the pressure on the pinched nerve is removed.

If you have any of the symptoms of a herniated disc mentioned above, this tells you that your disc is now pinching your nerve(s) and causing damage.

6 HOW NECK PAIN USUALLY STARTS AND HOW IT GETS WORSE

If we take things back one step further in figuring out the cause of your neck pain... you may be surprised to know that your neck pain may have started as abnormal movement or abnormal alignment of the bones in your spine... specifically in your neck.

This abnormal alignment and movement created uneven wear and tear on your spine... like the uneven wear and tear on your car tires when they're misaligned.

In the beginning, you may have noticed a clicking or a cracking sound when you moved your neck... especially in a certain direction. This is because the misaligned part of your spine was probably rubbing abnormally against other parts.

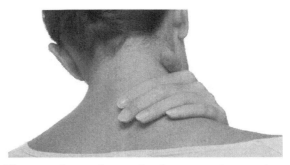

You may have also noticed your neck muscles feeling STIFF... especially in the morning.

You may have found yourself massaging your neck or trying to stretch your neck throughout the day.

**Studies suggest that the longer
your spinal misalignments go uncorrected,
the GREATER your risk.**

If your neck didn't get treated properly, it would have gotten worse.

Unfortunately, uncorrected spinal misalignments will usually advance to abnormal spinal conditions such as Spinal Arthritis, Bulged Discs or Herniated Discs, Degenerative Joint Disease or Spinal Stenosis.

Any of the above conditions can lead to severe neck pain and/or loss of muscle strength in your arms and hands.

Before developing severe neck pain or muscle loss, you may have felt a sharp pain, a dull ache or stiffness in your neck… for days, months or even years.

If your neck condition didn't get treated properly, your minor neck pain and stiffness may have progressed to a sharp shooting pain, burning pain or numbness down your arm, forearm or hand… a condition that tells you that you now have a PINCHED NERVE.

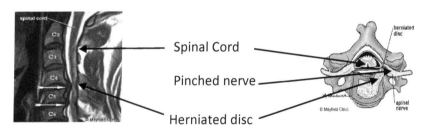

**Here's an example of a herniated disc in the neck.
In the picture on the right, notice the herniated disc pinching a nerve.**

Usually, arm and hand symptoms are only on one side. But, it's possible to have symptoms on both arms or hands.

For some people, their neck pain and/or arm/hand numbness and tingling comes and goes.

17

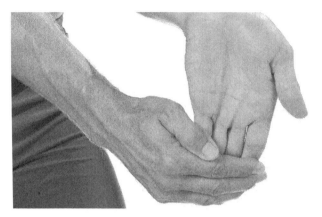

If you pay close attention, you'll notice that your pain, numbness or tingling is worse than the last episode.

In the beginning, your neck pain may have been more of an annoyance versus being debilitating. But your nerve pain and numbness can quickly become serious and debilitating after doing a MINOR activity such as sleeping the wrong way, sitting the wrong way, lifting an object... or after sneezing or coughing.

As your condition gets worse, your pinched nerve will slowly die.

Because of this, you'll lose function. Without proper nerve input, your hand, arm and forearm muscles on the side of your symptoms will get smaller and weaker.

Your affected muscles may also develop scar tissues... similar to the gristle that you see in a cheap cut of meat. Your lost muscle mass and lost muscle strength will make it more difficult for you to do your normal activities of daily living.

In the beginning, it's harder to notice your muscle loss.

Look at your arms, forearms and hands on both sides. Do you notice a difference in muscle mass between the two sides?

Also, if your neck pain and pinched nerve get worse, you may notice your muscles "giving way" while you do simple activities. When you get to this stage, you'll notice being more clumsy... for example, dropping things from your hand or spilling things more often.

18

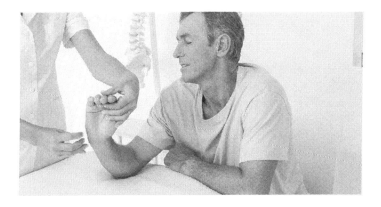

**Besides losing muscle mass and strength,
you'll also most likely LOSE
normal range of motion and flexibility
in your neck, arm, forearm and/or hand.**

A lot of people can deal with the nagging nerve pain or numbness… especially when it comes and goes. But it's a lot harder for people to deal with the loss of function that comes later when their neck pain or pinched nerve doesn't get fixed.

If caught and treated early, most neck pain can be fixed without much loss of function.

However, untreated neck pain that progresses to the advanced degenerative stages almost always results in PERMANENT loss of function that will affect your activities of daily living… including your job and your hobbies.

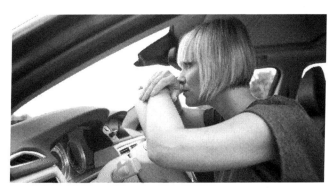

Driving can be excruciatingly painful… and dangerous for you.

The sooner you receive proper treatment for your neck pain, the better your chances of a FULL AND COMPLETE RECOVERY.

As soon as you feel that your neck pain is NOT going away... and getting WORSE... it's best if you consult a neck pain expert who can find the cause of your problem and help you get relief.

The earlier you seek treatment, the more options you have... and the less expensive it will be for you.

7 WHAT YOU SHOULD AVOID WHEN YOUR NECK HURTS

What exactly can you do to get neck pain relief?

You can get neck surgery... or you can try the following non-surgical ways to help you get neck pain relief... and hopefully help you avoid surgery for your neck

I have a chiropractic clinic in Soquel, CA. After 16 years in practice, I've helped over 3,500 patients and many of them suffered from neck pain.

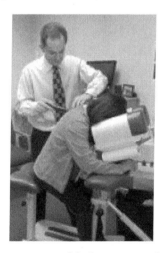

Here's an instrument-guided computerized treatment that I use on patients who don't want their necks cracked or twisted.

The advice that you're about to get are the same advice that I give to my patients who have neck pain.

Before you follow my suggestions below, be sure to consult with your doctor who is familiar with your medical history and current condition and get their okay. After you get their okay, here's what I advise you do...

First, let's STOP the DAMAGE.

If you have neck pain, here's the #1 neck position to AVOID: turning your head to one side... while looking down... while sneezing or coughing. You may even hear a "pop" in your neck when you injure your discs. This popping sound is *BAD NEWS*.

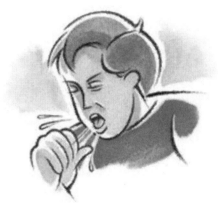

DON'T DO THIS...

Depending on how severe your condition is, doing this bad move can result in a herniated disc in your neck... or make your bulged or herniated disc much worse.

Many kids and adults do this without knowing how bad this position is for your neck. When you're young and limber, you may be able to assume this neck position without much pain afterward.

As you get older, you'll notice stiffness or pain in your neck after doing the above position... or soon after.

When you feel a sneeze or a cough coming... keep your head and neck in neutral position while you sneeze or cough. Neutral position meaning... looking straight ahead WITHOUT twisting your head to one side and

22

WITHOUT bending your head down.

Here are other things that you should AVOID...

Don't reach and/or lift an object from a position above your head. If the object that you're reaching for and lifting or pulling is heavy... your neck is in BIG TROUBLE. **You should also avoid the neck positions that make your neck pain worse.**

Take note of the activities that you do that require you to do the BAD combo move above... and either avoid these activities or change them.

When it comes to neck pain... NO pain, NO gain is NOT a good rule. Some people feel like the pain is creating a good stretch in their neck.

Not so... if you're putting your neck in a position that makes your neck pain worse, you're probably doing more HARM than GOOD.

Avoiding positions that make your neck pain worse is a simple RULE OF THUMB that you should follow. Following this rule of thumb will help relieve your pain and speed up your recovery.

Ignoring this rule of thumb, will make your neck pain worse and will make your neck pain treatment NOT as effective.

The painful neck positions to AVOID are different for different people.

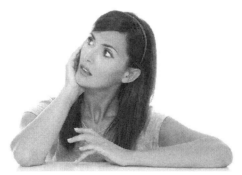

Depending on what the painful neck positions are for you... tells a neck pain expert A LOT about what may be wrong with your neck.

23

What about moving your neck in different positions to loosen it up? If done correctly, it's good to stretch and loosen up your neck. But, don't move your neck in the directions that cause pain… SHARP PAIN.

Another thing to avoid is sitting too long… especially with BAD POSTURE.

The chronic habit of sitting too long puts a lot of pressure on your neck muscles, ligaments and discs.

As much as possible, minimize your sitting time. But, this might be easier said than done. Maybe your job or daily life requires you to SIT for long periods of time.

If you absolutely have to sit for long periods during your waking hours, sit with proper posture… looking straight ahead… with your ears in line with your shoulders. I'll cover proper posture later in this book.

Also, make sure you have proper workstation set up at your job. Have an assessment to see if you have proper ergonomics while you work.

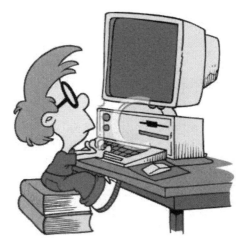

If you notice that your neck hurts at work, you may not have proper ergonomics.

When you're at work, be sure to take frequent breaks to rest your neck. Even if you do everything right, some jobs are NOT neck-friendly… so AVOID these jobs. One common mistake people make is doing jobs that are hard on the neck. These jobs make you prone to neck injuries... and you'll usually feel the damage you've done to your neck as you get older.

8 THE PROPER STANDING AND SITTING POSTURE FOR NECK PAIN RELIEF

Now that we've told you what neck positions to avoid... you should be wondering what the best neck position is. Let's now discuss proper neck and head posture.

According to Nobel Prize winner Dr. Hans Selye, M.D., *"The beginning of the disease process starts with postural distortions."* I'll expand on this later.

Have you ever noticed how many people have terrible posture? One of the most common faulty postures is called "forward head carriage" or "anterior weight bearing." Other terms are "hump back" or slouching. Thanks to cell phones and computers, this BAD posture is now common.

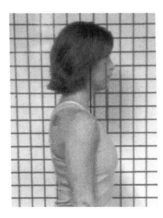

Do you hold your head forward in front of your shoulders like in the picture above?

26

With proper posture, your ear opening should be in line with your shoulder.

Have someone look at you from the side. <u>Is your head sitting straight above your neck and in line with your shoulders? Is your ear opening centrally aligned with your shoulders?</u>

If you do a lot of reading, desk work, computer work or driving, you are more likely to suffer from poor posture called Forward Head Carriage.

There are several reasons for this common postural fault. One reason is that muscles that attach to your skull have different degrees of strength. They also attach and pull at different angles, contributing to the common forward head carriage posture.

The muscles of the chest are MUCH STRONGER than those in the mid and upper back and tend to pull our shoulders forward.

Plus, a lot of Americans tend to look down a lot... reading, looking at their phone, working at their desk, etc... adding to the muscular discrepancy between the chest muscles and mid and upper back muscles.

Keep in mind that your head is HEAVY... especially if you're smart and talented and have a lot of brain mass. A lot of smart and talented people develop neck pain.

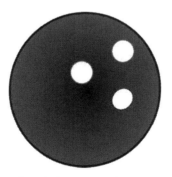

**An average head weighs approximately 10-13 pounds.
That's about the weight of a bowling ball.**

Also, <u>every inch your head pokes forward places an additional 10 lbs.</u> of load on your upper back muscles to keep your head upright. If your head

27

is positioned too far forward, the muscles in your upper back and neck tighten up much more than normal... these muscles become tired... and painful. Thus, you feel neck pain.

The picture below offers a good view of both a faulty posture as well as a "good" posture when standing.

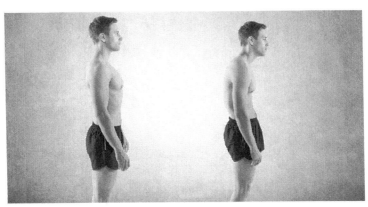

The picture on the left shows proper standing posture.
The picture on the right shows improper standing posture.

Besides being bad for your neck and shoulders, Forward Head Carriage and forward shoulders also constrict your heart and lungs. Over time, having less room for your heart and lungs will have a negative effect on your overall health.

You should correct these faulty postures as soon as possible.

It's important to understand that correcting Forward Head Carriage takes time – in fact, it takes a minimum of 3 months before this becomes an automatic new "habit."

Of course, it could take longer or, completely fail IF you are not VERY conscientious about CONSTANTLY reminding yourself to assume good sitting and standing posture.

Here's one exercise that you can do to correct your posture:

Look straight ahead. Retract your chin or head as far back as you can. Hold this position for 5-10 seconds. Do this multiple times a day to retrain your head to maintain a good posture.

28

This posture correction exercise will be either painful or difficult to do if you have joints in your neck and shoulders that are inflamed, misaligned or not moving properly... **or if you already have a pinched nerve or a herniated disc in your neck. If the above exercise is painful, get your neck condition treated first.**

Here's another comment on the importance of good posture:

Poor posture is associated with asymmetries in motion, leading to accelerated degenerative spinal joint pathology that will, in time, adversely affect the nervous system. (Koch et al, 2002)

Since we spend a lot of time sitting, what's the best sitting posture?

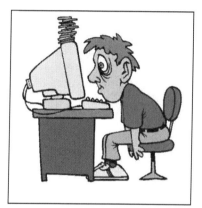

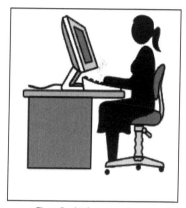

Bad sitting posture...   **Good sitting posture...**

To sit with good posture, put your head in neutral position... looking straight ahead... not looking up and not looking down. Make sure your head is in line with your neck, shoulders and low back. This is the best sitting posture.

Can you COMFORTABLY keep this position for 30 MINUTES?

If not, you most likely have a problem in your neck or low back that's preventing you from having good posture.

Good posture is not just good for your back... it's also good for the rest of your body... and for your overall health and well-being. Let me show you just how important good posture is to your health. Let's test how posture affects your lung capacity and LUNG HEALTH.

1. Sit on a chair.
2. Take a deep breath.
3. Assume the best posture position for your back.
4. Take a deep breath.
5. Now slouch as much as you can or assume a bad posture.
6. Take a deep breath.

Could you tell the difference between your lung's ability to get enough oxygen when you sit with a GOOD posture versus when you sit with a BAD posture?

Every part of your body relies on getting enough oxygen to stay healthy.. function well... and to NOT get DISEASE.

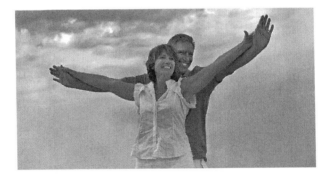

If you continue to sit or stand with a bad posture that minimizes the flow of oxygen to the rest of your body parts that need oxygen... it's just a matter of time before your oxygen-deprived body parts will break down... and disease will set in.

Here again is Dr. Selye's quote from the beginning of this chapter:

"The beginning of the disease process starts with postural distortions." This statement seems far-fetched at first. BUT... I hope you realize now that it makes sense. After all, Dr. Hans Selye, M.D. is a Nobel Prize winner. He MUST know what he's talking about.

9 WALK... WALK... WALK

Walking is one often overlooked activity that can relieve neck pain. Walking is ESSENTIAL to your healing and recovery... a simple yet powerful activity. Walking is a fantastic way to exercise your neck and back and make them strong and flexible.

Walk a few steps right now with your arms lightly swinging by your side. Did you feel your spinal muscles, ligaments and joints moving? You may not have felt your joints and ligaments moving, but you should have felt the muscles along your spine moving.

Try it again... and don't forget the gentle arm swing.

Walking creates a POWERFUL PUMP in your spine that helps pump fluids and nutrients in and out of your spinal joints... including your spinal discs.

Walking is a good way to maintain good circulation in your spine. Walking will also help prevent stiffness of your muscles and keep them from getting too spastic.

Also, if you pay close attention while you walk, you'll notice that your spinal muscles move in a synchronized way... where they alternate between stretching and contracting... a very elegant movement that's an absolute MUST for keeping your spinal muscles relaxed, flexible, strong and healthy.

31

Walk again... with a gentle arm swing... and see if you can feel this synchronized movement of your neck and back muscles. It may be harder to feel the movement of your neck muscles, but they move when you walk.

So, whenever you're able... WALK. But, don't overdo it. Too much of anything... including something that's good for you... is NOT good.

If you're like most people with neck pain, you're probably NOT walking too much. Squeeze in more walking time during your daily life to help relieve your neck pain.

If you're not used to walking... or if your neck pain is severe... you may have to start walking on FLAT, SOFT surfaces such as grass or trails first before you tackle walking on hills... or on a harder surface like pavement.

Also, if you're like most people with neck pain, you may be out of shape. You can even START walking inside your house. If you feel the need to rest or to sit down after walking a short distance... sit down and rest.

If you have someone you can walk with, walk with them. Walking with a partner is not only good for your back, but it will also be good for your emotional health.

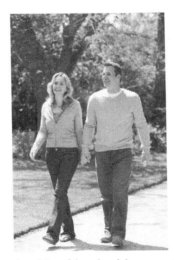

Take a healthy friend with you who can help you in case you need extra assistance.

If you're able, walk outside so that you can get the benefit of getting extra oxygen in your system. Oxygen is also VITAL to your healing and recovery.

Make sure there are rest stops along the way for you to sit on in case you need to rest.

If walking makes your neck pain unbearable, you should talk to your doctor for other things you can do to at least keep your lower back and legs moving.

If your doctor says that it's okay for you to do some walking, don't overdo it. Do not go beyond your pain tolerance. Do not go beyond your fitness tolerance.

10 HOW MUCH WATER YOU SHOULD DRINK FOR YOUR CONDITION

How much water is adequate? Do you need 8 glasses of water a day... no matter how tall you are or how much you weigh?

Here's a different suggestion as far as proper fluid intake that takes your body size and activity level into account.

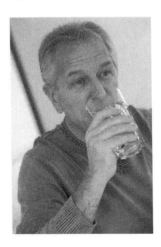

Divide your weight in half and the number you get is the amount of fluids in ounces (ozs.) that you should be drinking throughout the day.

For example, if you weigh 160 lbs... dividing 160 by 2 gives you 80...

so you should drink about 80 ounces of water a day.

If you're more active during the day, you may need more water that day. Also, if the weather is hot, you may need more water.

Making sure you get enough fluids will help you recover from neck pain. This is especially important for people with dehydrated spinal discs... which is often the case in people who suffer from neck pain.

Water also helps flush inflammatory byproducts out of your system.

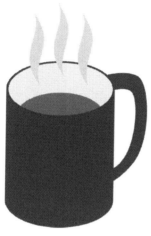

**Make sure you're drinking good quality fluids
and not the kind that dehydrate you
such as coffee, alcohol or sodas.**

Also, you might notice that when you drink more water, you tend to use the bathroom more. This is usual for most people in the beginning when they increase their water intake. Soon, your body should adjust to your new hydration level.

You may also need less water... especially if you don't have an active lifestyle. Too much of anything including something that's good for you such as water, is NOT good.

Get enough water, but not too much.

11 SHOULD YOU USE ICE OR HEAT FOR YOUR NECK PAIN?

Ice your neck to help relieve your neck pain. Ice is an anti-inflammatory agent... meaning it reduces inflammation or swelling.

Ice reduces congestion or PUSHES out of the injured area painful chemicals and fluids that build up when there's inflammation.

Ice usually feels good... once the part that you're icing is numb... but because ice is cold, it may not feel good in the beginning.

Heat does the opposite of ice.

Heat PULLS fluids INTO an area. Unlike ice, heat feels good initially. But... often, people who use heat on their neck say that it later made their neck problem WORSE. This is because the additional fluid build-up in an already inflamed or injured area is like throwing gasoline on a fire.

When using ice therapy... instead of using ice cubes, it's better to use the moldable ice packs like the ones with the gel-like material inside.

Choose the size of the ice pack carefully.

Depending on the size of your neck, you may not need such a big ice pack that makes your head and upper back numb. Use an ice pack that covers the base of your head and your upper shoulder area. If that's too cold for you, choose a smaller ice pack.

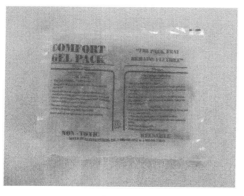

**These moldable ice packs come in different sizes and quality.
Part of your at-home first aid supply should be a good ice pack.**

Where *exactly* should you put the ice pack? Put the ice pack over the area of your neck that hurts... usually on the back of the neck. Be careful icing the sides and the front of your neck, since these areas have important structures under the skin that may be negatively affected by extreme cold.

DON'T PUT THE ICE PACK DIRECTLY ON YOUR SKIN.

Instead, put a thin piece of clothing... like your t-shirt... or a thin towel between your skin and the ice pack. You can have a thicker barrier if you're too chilled when using just a t-shirt or a thin towel.

Also, DO NOT lie face down. Instead, ice your neck while you're lying face up or while you're sitting.

And how long exactly should you keep the ice pack on?

This really depends on your current condition and diagnosis. If you have a condition that is "uncomplicated," use the ice pack for 15-20 minutes every 3-4 hours.

WARNING: Before you use ice, make sure you don't have a vascular or a neurologic condition that makes it unsafe for you to use ice.

12 THE NECK PAIN EXERCISES
THAT YOU SHOULD CONSIDER DOING

Neck stretching exercises work best when the cause of your neck pain is from a tight or spastic muscle.

PROCEED WITH CAUTION WITH THESE EXERCISES.

If you don't know exactly which neck stretches and exercises to do, DON'T do any. Ignorance in this area can hurt you and can make your neck pain worse

But... there are easy exercises that most people with neck pain can safely do. If you feel SHARP PAIN in your neck... or anywhere... while doing any of these exercises, STOP immediately.

Many neck problems can be relieved by neck exercises. But if you're getting SHARP PAIN with any of the exercises below, your neck pain may be beyond this point.

You may have a serious condition that needs expert help.

WARNING: As a general rule, if your neck pain is caused by a herniated disc or a bulged disc, DON'T do the exercises that require you to look up. If your condition is severe, you may not find a comfortable position... all positions may hurt.

Some of the exercises that I'll show you are advanced... so depending on how severe your neck pain is... you may not be able to do all of these.

Typically, when you do the exercises that are "BAD" for your specific condition, you'll notice that your neck pain, and/or arm, forearm or hand numbness and/or tingling will feel WORSE.

It's best to consult a neck pain expert who can help you determine the cause of your neck problem before you do any of these exercises.

There are 4 reasons to perform neck exercises:

1. Posture Correction
2. Stretch Tight Muscles
3. Strengthen Weak Or Injured Muscles
4. Coordination Of Neck Movement

POSTURE: The biggest culprit in this category is the Forward Head Carriage. If you look around a crowded airport, bus stop, train station, or mall, you can see MANY examples of this.

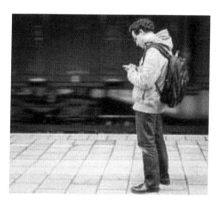

**This faulty posture is estimated to occur
in 66-90% of the population.**

Also, forward head posture is STRONGLY associated with decreased respiratory muscle strength, which <u>can reduce lung capacity and our ability to breathe by as much as 30%!</u>

It's also linked to tension headaches, altered eye and ear function, high blood pressure, and over time it can lead to arthritis, herniated discs, pinched nerves, and more.

The "classic" appearance is that position of the head is too far forward, the shoulders roll forward and the upper back sticks out.

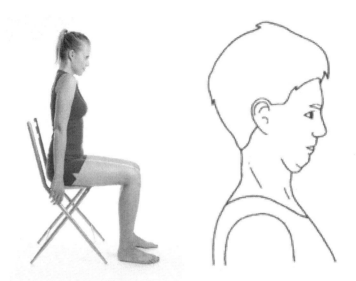

Here's one exercise that may help improve your posture:

1. Look straight ahead. Tighten your core by performing an abdominal brace. This is done by contracting your belly muscles so that when you poke your thumbs into your sides and front, you feel a firm abdominal muscle wall. You don't have to "brace" at a 100% of maximum. Shoot for 25-50% or just enough to feel the muscles contract. Relax and contract several times so you're sure you can feel the muscles tighten up. Keep a curve in your lower back when you do this... and don't slouch.

2. Lift your chest. This will improve the rounded shoulders and slouched upper back posture. Think of lifting your chest towards the ceiling more than just sticking it out.

3. Perform chin retractions – do 10 retractions every hour. Set the timer on your cell phone to remind you. Do this gently, slowly, and to a firm end-point of movement. If you feel like you are creating a "double or triple chin," you're doing it right.

This a GREAT way to "re-program" your nervous system and when you find yourself doing this WITHOUT THINKING, it will have become a new... and good... habit.

STRETCHING: Since our neck muscles have to hold up our 12 lb. head, it's no wonder our neck muscles seem to be tight almost all the time.

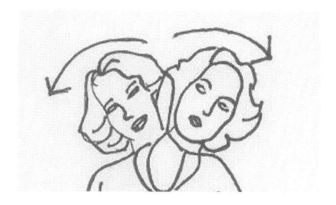

Below are stretching exercises for your neck:

1. Drop your chin to your chest
2. Look at the ceiling
3. Turn your head to the left, then to right
4. Touch your ear to your shoulder…without shoulder shrugging. Do this on both sides.

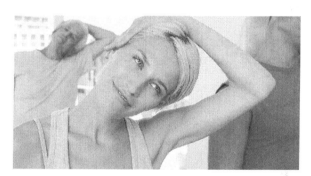

Here's a combo stretch for neck pain that's fast and efficient.

Bend your head to the right… while reaching over the left side of your head with your right hand… and gently pulling on your head until you feel a gentle stretch on the left side of your neck. Now reach down with your opposite hand (left hand)… as if there's a dollar bill on the ground and you can't quite reach it. If you overdo this, the side(s) of your neck will be sore.

While doing the above stretch, tuck in your chin… drop your head forward… and backward… and turn your head a little from side to side to gently stretch different tight muscle fibers.

Repeat on the opposite side. This stretch can be done while sitting or standing. Do this stretch multiple times a day, especially when your neck feels tight – like after doing computer work, for example.

STRENGTHENING: Most people have Forward Head Carriage. The farther forward the head sits, the greater the load on the muscles in the back of the neck and upper back to hold it up.

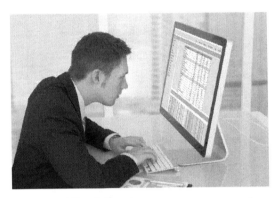

This Forward Head Carriage creates a negative spiral or "vicious cycle" that can lead to many complaints.

Problems you may develop from this bad posture include... but not limited to... neck pain, headaches, balance disturbances... and in the long-term... osteoarthritis.

If you have Forward Head Carriage, you have two important groups of muscles that require strengthening: your deep neck flexors and deep neck extensors.

The deep neck flexors are muscles located directly on the front of the cervical spine or neck. These muscles are described as being "involuntary" or unable to be voluntarily contracted.

Therefore, we have to "trick" the voluntary outer "extrinsic" (stronger) muscles into NOT WORKING so that your deep, intrinsic ones will contract and get stronger.

Be careful with the exercises that I'm about to show you. If they hurt, DON'T do them.

Flex your chin to your chest and push your neck... not your head... back over your shoulders into resistance caused a towel wrapped around the back of your neck.

42

For this exercise, if you feel your chin raise towards the ceiling, you're doing it WRONG!

Keep your chin tucked as close to your chest as possible as you push your neck... not your head... backward. If you're doing it correctly, your chest should raise towards the ceiling as you push your chin down and neck back.

The deep neck extensors are strengthened in a very similar way, EXCEPT here you DO push the back of your HEAD back into your towel while keeping your chin tucked tightly into your chest.

COORDINATION: Coordination-based exercises are important because they stimulate our neuro-motor system and can help restore normal function.

To increase your coordination, you can make simple exercises more complex. For example, you can do your neck exercises while you sit on an exercise ball. This will enhance your proprioception and will increase your overall coordination and balance. Be careful if you have problems with balance and/or dizziness.

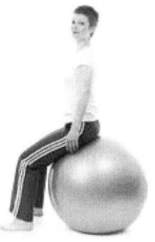

**Before you add an exercise ball to your routine,
make sure you're comfortable doing the exercises without the ball.**

Another way to enhance your coordination is to add resistance to your neck stretching and strengthening exercises.

For example, when you're done with the exercise, release slowly... and keep resisting.

If you apply resistance while your muscles elongate... this "eccentric resistance" will help you build COORDINATION. If you apply resistance while your muscles contract... this "concentric resistance" will help you build STRENGTH.

Using your hand, only use a light amount of resistance when exercising your neck muscles... only 10% - 20% of maximum push. Your head and your hand will "arm wrestle" with each other.

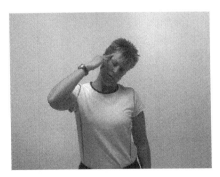 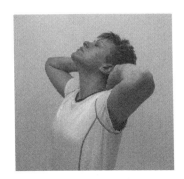

Do the stretching exercises for the neck that I covered earlier in this chapter. For each range of motion... let your hand win... and then let your head win.

The trick is to do these exercises VERY slowly... to build motor control and coordination. Also, move slowly through the entire "comfortable" range of motion. If your neck pain gets worse, lighten up on the amount of pressure used... or stop the movement just prior to the sharp pain onset.

With all of the neck exercises and stretches that I discussed in this section, you're probably asking the following questions:

- How long should I hold each position?
- How many repetitions should I do?
- How many times a day should I do them?
- When should I do these exercises?

Let's start with how long you should hold each position. Start holding each position for 2-3 seconds. As you get stronger, you may be able to hold them longer... but don't overdo it.

How many repetitions should you do?

Do as many as you can comfortably handle... and again, don't overdo it! Start with 3-5 reps... less if you're not able to.

How many times a day should you do them?

Twice a day works well for most people. Also, it's best to do these exercises more often rather than do a lot of reps and/or long holds.

After you do the above exercises and stretches, you might feel sore in certain areas. Ice these areas... follow the icing instructions covered in the previous section.

When's the best time to do these exercises?

Do them at a time that works best for you. Also, they're so simple that if you feel your neck starting to hurt or starting to tighten up... stop what you're doing and do these exercises.

DON'T do these exercises first thing in the morning. Your muscles and ligaments won't be warmed up... you'll be more prone to injury.

Also, don't do these exercises when you're EXHAUSTED... your muscles and ligaments won't have as much strength to protect your joints if you overstretch.

13 HOW TO KEEP YOUR SPINE ALIGNED AND MOVING PROPERLY

Since misaligned spinal joints and/or spinal joints that don't move properly can cause neck pain… or make neck pain worse… make sure to keep your proper spinal alignment and motion.

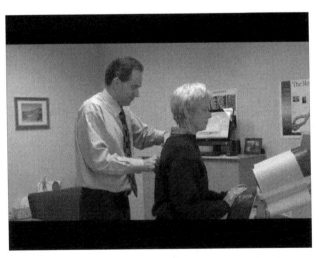

You should see a chiropractor who can check your spine for proper alignment and motion.

This will not only help relieve your neck pain, but keeping your spinal bones and joints aligned and moving properly will help prevent future problems from showing up later.

How?

Each bone and joint in your spine is connected to each other… especially the ones directly above and directly below each spinal bone/joint.

When you have spinal misalignment or abnormal spinal motion, the joints above and below the problem joint will need to compensate to keep the alignment and motion of your spine as close to normal as possible.

These joints will start to have problems if they have to keep compensating… then the bones and joints around them will also need to compensate causing problems in these areas.

If not stopped, you'll have a vicious cycle of spinal joint degeneration happening up and down your spine. You may notice that over time, the joints above and below the initial problem area will also develop degenerative joint problems.

This is why people with neck problems often also end up experiencing low back problems.

Different chiropractors use different chiropractic treatment techniques and different approaches to keep your spinal bones aligned and your spinal joints moving properly.

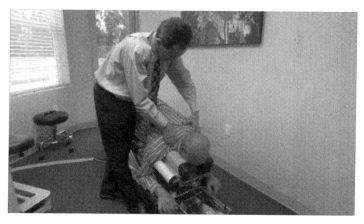

Some chiropractors use traditional hands-on treatments like this one above that I use at my clinic.

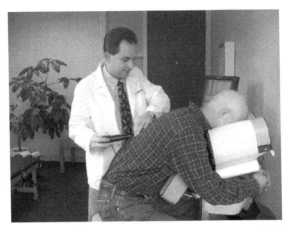

Some chiropractors use instrument-guided treatment like the one above. I use this on my patients who don't like their necks or backs cracked, popped or twisted.

The computerized spinal treatment pictured above uses a piezoelectric sensor to measure spinal joint motion. This sensor is attached to a mechanical stylus.

Both the sensor and the stylus are attached to a computer with a sophisticated software that's able to measure joint motion... and also able to calculate the amount of force needed to restore proper joint motion.

While the patient sits comfortably, I guide the sensor and the stylus up and down the patient's spine.

The sensor detects fixated spinal joints and the stylus unlocks the joint... and restores proper joint motion. How? The stylus gently oscillates up to 12 impulses per second. While the stylus oscillates, the sensor constantly monitors the joint's motion. When normal joint motion is restored, the oscillation stops.

How does this computerized spinal treatment decrease neck pain?

To review basic neurology, types 1, 2 and 3 neuronal fibers inhibit type 4 pain fibers. If a spinal joint is fixated or not moving properly, types 1,2 and 3 fibers are inhibited. This makes type 4 pain fibers fire more. This results in more neck pain for the patient. When this treatment restores normal spinal joint motion, types 1,2 and 3 fibers fire more. This inhibits the type 4 pain fibers. This is why patients feel relief of their neck pain after this treatment.

There are other instrument-guided treatments used by chiropractors. I prefer this one, because it's specific, scientific and precise. Not that other methods aren't. Also, my patients get great results with this treatment.

During this treatment, the patient remains fully clothed and comfortable. The whole treatment takes about 5-10 minutes. With this treatment, there's no need to crack or twist the patient's spine. Some patients prefer this method over the traditional chiropractic treatments.

Some of my patients prefer the traditional hands-on chiropractic treatments and that's what I use on them.

Both the traditional chiropractic treatments and the instrument-guided treatments work well. It's just a matter of my patient's comfort level and their preferred treatment method.

Find a chiropractor who uses a treatment style that works best for you.

Spinal joint problems and spinal misalignments are easy to treat and correct... especially when caught early. If left uncorrected, problems will eventually create a giant pain in the neck for you... like a cavity that's allowed to get much bigger and worse.

14 NECK PAIN TREATMENT OPTIONS

If you have neck pain, you have different treatment options. You can seek treatment from your primary doctor. The primary doctor's approach to neck pain management usually results in a prescription that may include an anti-inflammatory drug… and/or a muscle relaxant… and/or a painkiller.

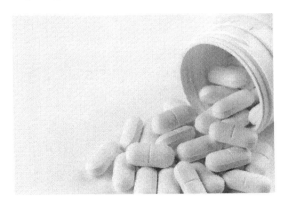

Some patients with simple and uncomplicated neck pain find relief with these medications. Some only find temporary relief of their neck pain… some don't get relief at all.

Also, some people with neck pain can't take these medications, because they have adverse side effects that they don't want or can't handle… and/or they're already taking medications that can't be mixed with these new ones for their neck pain.

Your doctor may also prescribe a series of physical therapy treatments. Some benefit from these treatments, some don't.

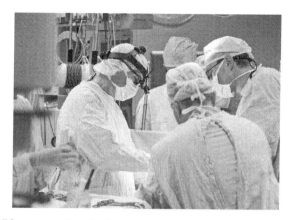

**If your neck pain has gotten progressively worse
with neurological loss and/or severe functional limitation,
your doctor may suggest a consult with a surgeon for neck surgery.**

In general, guidelines for treating neck pain that radiates into an arm recommend that patients undergo a course of "conservative"... or non-surgical care... FIRST before getting surgery. In fact, many guidelines DON'T even recommend MRI or EMG/NCV initially unless the result from the non-surgical care is not satisfactory.

Studies have shown that patients with neck and arm pain... most commonly caused by herniated discs... are frequently successfully managed WITHOUT SURGERY.

Therefore, a non-surgical approach like chiropractic care should be tried FIRST and surgery be reserved ONLY to the people who don't get good results from non-surgical treatments.

Other treatments for neck pain include injections, massage, acupuncture, etc.

How do you decide which treatment to choose?

Here's a look at 3 studies that compared 3 popular forms of care for chronic spinal pain... which includes neck pain. The study wanted to determine the short-term and more importantly, the LONG-TERM benefits of treatment.

The 3 treatments evaluated were: chiropractic treatment, acupuncture, and non-steroid anti-inflammatory drugs - NSAIDs like Advil.

Study #1: This study included a pilot group of 77 patients complaining of chronic spinal pain (neck, mid-back, or low-back pain). These patients were separated into one of the three treatment groups and received either NSAIDs, acupuncture, or chiropractic treatment. Patients received care for four weeks with outcome measures (questionnaires) used to assess changes in pain and disability.

After a 30-day time frame, only patients who received chiropractic care reached a level of statistically significant improvement, supporting chiropractic care to offer the best SHORT-TERM BENEFITS for those with chronic back/neck pain.

Study #2: This study included 115 patients, again randomized, to receive either one of the same three treatments... this time, the data was gathered two, five, and nine weeks after the start of treatment. Again, those who received chiropractic care experienced the best overall improvement at nine weeks.

Study #3: This study involved follow-up from the same patient group from the SECOND study two years later. Once again, participants completed outcome assessments that measure pain and disability. This time, the results showed that only the patients in the chiropractic care group maintained long-term improvement in pain and disability.

Many doctors now incorporate chiropractic care as part of their approach to managing neck pain, because it's safe, beneficial and cost-effective.

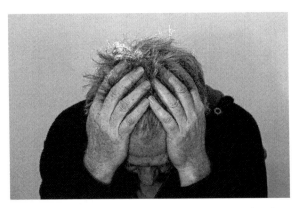

Most of my patients with neck come in because they've tried the other treatments and they still have neck pain... and their condition is getting worse... now affecting their sleep, daily life and work.

Neck pain is usually cost by a physical problem in the spine… most common is a fixated joint in the neck that needs to move normal again.

Traditionally, "rest and heat" are commonly prescribed for neck pain patients.

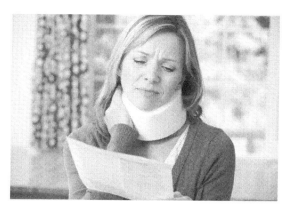

Sometimes, patients with neck pain are placed in a cervical collar and taken off work and told to rest.

If there's severe neck instability, this might be necessary. However, if there isn't, the evidence published STRONGLY disagrees with this approach… favoring a treatment plan that incorporates motion, gently getting back to "usual" activity… including work… chiropractic treatment… and exercise as soon as possible.

Each of the neck pain treatments that I mentioned above have their pros and cons. Each can be beneficial depending on what exactly is causing your neck pain.

One of the reasons why chiropractic treatment for neck pain works great is because we are using a physical form of treatment to unlock the problematic joint.

This in turn shuts off the signals from the joint to the brain… shutting off the protective muscle spasms. Sometimes, the improvement is immediate, but more often, several treatments may be required to complete the task.

In general, the recovery time is shorter the closer to the time of injury you are treated, so getting prompt treatment is very important. I also recommend that my patients do the neck exercises and at-home treatments that I covered in this book. These further speed up their recovery time.

Some people with neck pain refuse to seek the help of a chiropractor. They've heard that once you go to a chiropractor, you have to keep going for life. Different chiropractors have different treatment techniques and different office policies.

At my clinic, I offer short-term chiropractic care. I have a very busy clinic. My goal with each of my patients is to get them better and out of my office as fast as possible.

If my patients get injured and/or if their symptoms return, they call my office to schedule a treatment. I don't put patients on long-term treatment plans… they call me when they need my help.

If you have neck pain, don't put off getting chiropractic treatment. Don't let your neck become ARTHRITIC.

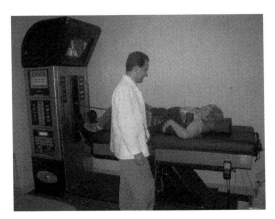

**Find a chiropractor that works well with
your preferences and get the help that you need.**

The sooner you get the help that you need, the better your prognosis… or outcome.

In the previous chapter, I've covered the chiropractic treatment methods that I use to keep my patients' spines aligned and moving properly… relieving their neck pain.

There are other treatments in my office that I use on my patients with neck pain. I want to tell you about one particular treatment that gets great results on my neck pain patients with radiating pain/tingling/numbness down their shoulder, arm, or hand.

This treatment is mechanical cervical traction. If your neck pain or pinched nerve is from a bulged disc or a herniated disc, this treatment will gently stretch your neck... and decrease the pressure on your pinched nerves or nerve roots.

Be careful when trying neck stretching machines on your own. Some may help you. Some may make your condition worse. Be very careful with these at-home back stretching devices.

You may do more harm than good. Consult your doctor before trying one of these at-home devices.

No matter what neck pain treatment or device you try... don't lose hope. Many people with neck pain have successfully overcome their condition... or at least made their neck pain manageable without much loss of function... allowing them to continue to work and/or continue to enjoy their favorite activities and hobbies.

Aren't you tired of constantly trying to find a comfortable pain-free position? Have you LIMITED your activities to avoid getting seriously hurt?

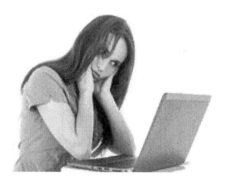

Is it getting harder to deal with your neck pain?
You probably lost so much function and flexibility already.

How much more flexibility and function can you stand to lose? You may have decided to live with your neck pain or your shoulder/arm/hand pain or numbness. After treating hundreds of patients with neck pain, I know that neck pain can progress from a manageable pain to a painfully debilitating pain… sometimes overnight.

After accidentally bending or twisting your neck in the "wrong direction," you may feel that instant knife stabbing pain in your neck, shoulder, arm or hand… compounded by a severe neck muscle spasm… that feels like a giant wrench clamping your neck… freezing you in your tracks… while your blood pressure and pulse rate skyrocket.

Get help now before this happens to you.

If after you follow the advice that I laid out in this book, your neck pain is not MUCH BETTER… you may have a condition that's beyond something that you can correct at home.

There are a lot of good doctors around that can help you with your neck pain. If you live in Santa Cruz County, California… or if you find yourself in this area, come by my clinic… The Back Pain And Sciatica Clinic… to see if I can help you with your neck pain. Below is my contact information:

Back Pain And Sciatica Clinic
Dr. John Falkenroth, D.C.
2959 Park Ave., Suite F
Soquel, CA 95073
(831) 475-8600
www.BackPainAndSciaticaClinic.com

I hope that the information that I shared with you will help relieve your neck pain. I wish you the best of luck in finding the neck pain relief that you're looking for.

Thank you for your time.

ABOUT THE AUTHOR

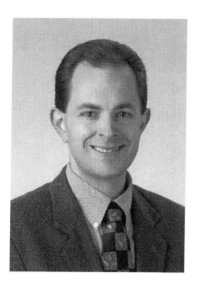

Dr. John Falkenroth, D.C. is the Clinic Director at the Back Pain And Sciatica Clinic in Soquel, California, USA. After over 15 years practicing chiropractic, Dr. Falkenroth has helped over 3,500 patients… many of them suffered from back pain, neck pain and sciatica.

Prior to attending chiropractic school, Dr. Falkenroth attended the University of California at Davis… where he earned a Bachelor of Science degree in Physiology in 1994.

While studying human physiology at the University of California at Davis, Dr. Falkenroth realized that pressure or impingement on the spinal nerve roots that exit the spine can negatively affect a person's health.

With this realization, Dr. Falkenroth decided to help others by becoming an expert in treating back pain, neck pain and sciatica.

To complement his excellent physiology background from UC Davis, Dr. Falkenroth decided to go to Davenport, Iowa, USA to attend the 100+ year old top-rated chiropractic college in the world – Palmer College – where he graduated *summa cum laude*.

Go to www.BackPainAndSciaticaClinic.com for more neck pain relief tips. You can also call Dr. Falkenroth's office at (831) 475-8600.

35951768R00038

Made in the USA
San Bernardino, CA
08 July 2016